BARBARA O'NEILL'S LOST ALKALINE REMEDY BIBLE

The Lost Remedies of Nature
for Contemporary Illnesses

Davila O'Neill MD

About the Author: Davila O'Neill

Davila O'Neill is a dedicated nutritionist and medical practitioner with over 15 years of experience in promoting healthful living. A graduate of California State University, Northridge, O'Neill brings a wealth of knowledge and expertise to the field of nutrition and natural health. With a deep passion for helping individuals achieve optimal well-being through balanced nutrition and holistic practices, O'Neill's work emphasizes practical, science-backed approaches to health. Her commitment to empowering others to live vibrant, healthy lives is reflected in her approachable writing and compassionate approach to wellness.

Table of Contents

INTRODUCTION 7

The Healing Power of Nature 7

Barbara O'Neill's Herbal Philosophy 7

The History and Resurgence of Natural Remedies 9

Why Natural Remedies Matter in Today's World 12

Holistic Healing Approach 13

Accessibility and Affordability 14

Fewer Side Effects 15

Environmental Impact and Sustainability 15

Aligning with Preventive Health 16

Respect for Cultural and Traditional Knowledge 17

Personal Empowerment and Connection to Nature.17

Rediscovering the Healing Power of Nature 18

CHAPTER ONE 21

The Fundamentals of Herbal Medicine 21

Common Types of Herbal Remedies and Their
Applications 23

Teas (Infusions and Decoctions) 23

Tinctures 23

Salves and Balms 24

Capsules and Powders 24

Essential Oils 25

Getting Started with Herbs 25

How to Source and Prepare Herbs Safely 25

Essential Equipment and Storage Techniques 27

Key Terms in Herbalism 28

The Science of Plant-Based Healing 29

How Herbs Interact with the Body 29

Alkaloids...29

Speed of Effectiveness 32

Side Effects and Safety......................................33

Sustainability and Accessibility 33

The Essentials for Herbal Healing 34

CHAPTER TWO 35

Essential Herbs for Everyday Health 35

Herbs for Specific Ailments...............................39

Herbal Remedies for Immune Support 39

Herbal Remedies for Digestion 40

Herbal Remedies for Stress and Anxiety...................41

Herbal Remedies for Sleep 42

Rare and Lost Remedies..43

Herbs with Historical Significance..........................43

Reviving Ancient Practices for Modern Benefits.......44

Safety and Contraindications for Common Herbs 45

Guidelines for Safe Use...46

Rediscovering Plant-Based Healing for Modern
Wellness..47

CHAPTER THREE 48

Preparing and Using Herbal Remedies 48

Herbal Teas and Tinctures 48

Decoction Method (For Roots and Bark) 50

Tincture-Making for Concentrated Herbal Extracts..51

Basic Tincture Recipe 51

Balms, Salves, and Ointments..................................52

Basic Ingredients for Topical Remedies 53

Making the Balm or Salve 54

Natural Tonics and Elixirs..56

Everyday Tonics for Vitality and Immune Support ...56

Building Routines for Wellness with Tonics and Elixirs
....59

Embracing Herbal Remedies in Daily Life 60

CHAPTER FOUR 61

Herbal strategies for stress relief, sleep improvement,
and mental clarity...61

Immune System Boosters 61

Herbs to Strengthen and Maintain Immune Health .62

Seasonal Immunity Tips 64

Respiratory and Cardiovascular Support 64

Herbs for Respiratory Health 65

Herbs for Heart Wellness..66

Remedies for Colds, Flu, and Respiratory Ailments ..67

Herbal Aids for Digestion 68

Herbs for Liver Health..69

Stress, Sleep, and Mental Wellness 70

Herbal Strategies for Stress Relief 70

Herbs for Sleep Improvement...................................72

Herbs for Mental Clarity 72

Herbal Routines for Mental Wellness........................73

CHAPTER FIVE 75

Barbara's Legacy of Herbal Wisdom 75

The Future of Herbal Medicine..................................75

Where Herbal Medicine is Heading in the Modern Era
....75

Integrating Herbal Remedies into Your Life
Responsibly 77

Herbal Gardening and Sustainable Harvesting 78

How to Grow, Harvest, and Sustainably Source Herbs
....78

Building Your Own Herbal Garden at Home 80

Sharing Herbal Knowledge with Others....................82

Building a Legacy of Health through Natural Remedies
....83

Appendices 86

Glossary of Herbal Terms...............................87

The Healing Power of Nature

Barbara O'Neill's Herbal Philosophy

Barbara O'Neill is celebrated for her deep commitment to promoting natural healing through herbal remedies, a dedication that draws from both tradition and modern understanding of plant-based treatments. Her approach centers around the belief that nature has provided all we need to support our health, offering potent, effective remedies for various ailments that are often less invasive and more sustainable than many pharmaceutical treatments. O'Neill's philosophy is rooted in the principles of holistic health, emphasizing the need to treat the body, mind, and spirit as an interconnected system rather than addressing symptoms in isolation.

For Barbara O'Neill, the use of herbal remedies is not merely an alternative to conventional medicine; it is a lifestyle choice that aligns with respecting the natural world and understanding our place within it. She encourages using plants responsibly and sustainably, appreciating the power that herbs can bring to our lives. According to O'Neill, herbalism is not just about "fixing" health problems; it's about achieving harmony between the body and its environment, supporting the body's own natural healing processes, and building resilience to illness.

O'Neill also emphasizes education and self-empowerment. She advocates for individuals to learn about herbs, understand their properties, and develop a sense of confidence in using them for self-care. Her philosophy underscores that everyone should have access to knowledge about the natural world and how to harness its healing potential.

Barbara's teachings encourage her followers to look beyond symptomatic relief, encouraging deeper awareness of lifestyle choices, diet, and preventive care as essential components of a healthy, balanced life. This integrative approach where herbal knowledge is combined with lifestyle changes embodies a core part of her herbal philosophy.

The History and Resurgence of Natural Remedies

Herbal medicine is one of the oldest forms of healing, with roots that extend back thousands of years across cultures worldwide. Ancient texts from civilizations such as Mesopotamia, Egypt, China, and India contain descriptions of medicinal plants, many of which remain popular in modern herbalism.

In traditional Chinese medicine (TCM), Ayurvedic medicine, and Indigenous healing practices across the Americas, Africa, and Europe, plants were foundational to health care systems, each culture developing an extensive pharmacopeia.

In these early societies, the use of plants was not purely functional but often symbolic and spiritual. Many herbs were associated with specific gods, seasons, or energies, and their use extended beyond physical healing to rituals, spiritual ceremonies, and cultural rites of passage. This holistic, interconnected perspective of health has carried forward into today's herbal practices, continuing to emphasize the need to address the physical, emotional, and spiritual dimensions of well-being.

In the West, the knowledge of herbal remedies was passed down through generations until the Industrial Revolution, which brought rapid advances in chemistry and pharmacology.

These scientific breakthroughs shifted focus towards synthesized compounds and standardized pharmaceutical drugs. By the early 20th century, many traditional herbal practices were overshadowed or discredited, considered "folk medicine" rather than legitimate science. However, this trend also created a rift between synthetic medications, which often focus on quick, targeted results, and traditional plant medicines, which are generally slower acting and address the root causes of imbalance.

Despite this shift, herbal medicine persisted as an "alternative" form of healing, sustained by holistic health practitioners and Indigenous communities who maintained their traditional practices. In recent decades, herbal remedies have enjoyed a resurgence in popularity, driven by growing awareness of the limitations of conventional medicine, interest in natural and sustainable living, and scientific research that has validated the efficacy of many medicinal plants. Studies on herbs like turmeric, echinacea, and St.

John's wort, for instance, have demonstrated their effectiveness for inflammation, immune support, and mental health, respectively, leading to a renewed respect for plant-based healing.

This revival has sparked a renewed interest in learning from ancient healing systems. Today, herbalism is again embraced by many as part of a lifestyle focused on prevention and wellness rather than disease management alone. People are seeking alternatives to the sometimes harsh side effects of pharmaceuticals, and many are turning to natural remedies to help manage chronic illnesses and enhance their overall well-being.

Why Natural Remedies Matter in Today's World

In an era where rapid industrialization and technological advances have transformed every aspect of life, the resurgence of natural remedies reflects a growing desire to reconnect with the natural world.

In modern society, health issues such as chronic stress, pollution, and processed foods have led to an epidemic of lifestyle-related diseases, including obesity, diabetes, and heart disease. These conditions often require long-term treatment plans, which can be costly and may involve medications with adverse side effects. Natural remedies offer an alternative approach that addresses not only the symptoms but also the underlying causes of these modern ailments.

Holistic Healing Approach

Unlike pharmaceutical medications that are designed to target specific symptoms or processes, herbal remedies offer a holistic approach to health. Many herbs, such as adaptogens, can help balance bodily functions, supporting overall resilience rather than addressing a single ailment.

Herbs like ashwagandha, reishi, and holy basil, for example, help regulate the body's response to stress, promoting mental and emotional balance while simultaneously strengthening the immune system and enhancing physical endurance. This multi-faceted approach aligns with the understanding that health is dynamic and interconnected.

Accessibility and Affordability

Herbal remedies provide accessible and affordable options for individuals around the world. While pharmaceuticals can be prohibitively expensive, especially in countries without adequate healthcare systems, many herbal options are comparatively low-cost and can even be grown at home. Herbs like chamomile, peppermint, and aloe vera are relatively easy to cultivate and offer a range of benefits from calming digestive upsets to soothing burns.

Encouraging self-sufficiency and knowledge of local plants, herbalism empowers people to take control of their health.

Fewer Side Effects

Although any potent remedy must be used with care, herbs generally have fewer side effects than synthetic medications. Because herbs are complex mixtures of compounds rather than single-molecule drugs, their effects are usually more balanced and less likely to cause dramatic side effects. For example, while non-steroidal anti-inflammatory drugs (NSAIDs) are commonly used for pain relief, they often cause gastrointestinal issues with prolonged use. In contrast, herbs like turmeric and ginger offer natural anti-inflammatory benefits with far fewer risks.

Environmental Impact and Sustainability

The modern pharmaceutical industry relies on a high level of industrial production, which can be damaging to the environment.

Manufacturing drugs involves synthetic chemicals and extensive energy use, often leaving behind a significant carbon footprint. Herbal remedies, on the other hand, have a smaller environmental impact, particularly when plants are cultivated sustainably. Growing medicinal plants encourages biodiversity, and small-scale herbal production is often integrated with organic farming practices. By choosing natural remedies, people contribute to a more sustainable and ecologically responsible form of healthcare.

Aligning with Preventive Health

Herbalism is inherently preventive in nature, supporting wellness practices that can ward off disease. Many herbs are rich in antioxidants, vitamins, and minerals that help boost immunity and protect against cellular damage. For instance, elderberry and echinacea are known for their immune-boosting properties and are widely used during flu season to prevent or reduce the severity of respiratory illnesses.

Rather than waiting until an ailment arises, using herbs as part of daily health maintenance supports long-term resilience and reduces the need for invasive treatments.

Respect for Cultural and Traditional Knowledge

The rediscovery of herbal remedies in modern contexts has sparked a renewed respect for Indigenous and traditional knowledge. Many Indigenous communities have a deep understanding of the plants native to their regions, and their wisdom offers valuable insights into sustainable, respectful practices for using these plants. By embracing herbal remedies, we can recognize and honor the knowledge of these cultures, promoting ethical and respectful sharing of knowledge.

Personal Empowerment and Connection to Nature

Herbal remedies encourage individuals to take an active role in their own health.

Growing, harvesting, and preparing herbs is a grounding practice that can enhance one's connection to nature. Learning about herbs promotes a sense of empowerment and self-reliance, as people acquire practical skills to care for themselves and their families. This personal empowerment goes hand-in-hand with environmental stewardship, as people who feel connected to nature are more likely to advocate for sustainable practices and protect the environment.

Rediscovering the Healing Power of Nature

The resurgence of herbal remedies signals a return to simplicity and a reminder that, despite technological advancements, nature's wisdom remains relevant. By embracing herbalism, we not only tap into ancient knowledge but also discover a more sustainable, gentle way to care for our health.

As Barbara O'Neill emphasizes in her philosophy, natural remedies offer us the opportunity to work with the body, not against it, fostering a sense of balance and well-being that modern medicine often overlooks.

In today's world, where healthcare systems face immense strain, and people seek alternatives to synthetic drugs, the healing power of nature offers hope and inspiration. Herbs reconnect us with a slower, more mindful approach to wellness, where prevention and self-care are paramount. In the pages that follow, Barbara O'Neill's Lost Bible of Herbal Remedies will guide you through this journey of rediscovering nature's cures, empowering you to take control of your health in a way that is natural, sustainable, and deeply enriching.

This introduction sets the stage by delving into Barbara O'Neill's philosophy, the historical and cultural significance of herbal medicine, and the reasons why natural remedies are particularly valuable in today's world. Let me know if you need further adjustments to fit your vision for the book!

CHAPTER ONE

The Fundamentals of Herbal Medicine

Basics of Herbal Medicine and Holistic Health.

Herbal medicine, also known as phytotherapy, is the practice of using plants and plant extracts to promote healing and maintain wellness. It is a discipline with roots in ancient healing traditions from around the world, such as Traditional Chinese Medicine (TCM), Ayurveda, and Indigenous practices across various cultures. Unlike conventional medicine, which often focuses on symptom management, herbal medicine aligns more with holistic health principles, addressing the mind, body, and spirit as an integrated system.

Holistic health emphasizes the concept that the body has an innate ability to heal when given the right support.

Herbal remedies act as allies, supporting the body in achieving balance or "homeostasis," which is essential for maintaining health. For example, adaptogens, a group of herbs like ashwagandha and rhodiola, are known for their ability to help the body adapt to stress, improving resilience and aiding in mental clarity. Similarly, bitter herbs such as dandelion and gentian support digestive health by stimulating bile production and aiding digestion, a critical aspect of holistic wellness.

Holistic health also considers the mental and emotional aspects of healing. Herbs like chamomile, lavender, and valerian are not only helpful for calming the nervous system but also promote emotional well-being. By focusing on holistic health, herbal medicine encourages us to look beyond individual symptoms and address underlying imbalances that may contribute to illness.

Common Types of Herbal Remedies and Their Applications

Herbal medicine encompasses various forms of remedies, each prepared in a way that maximizes the benefits of the plant. Some of the most common types of herbal remedies include:

Teas (Infusions and Decoctions)

Teas are one of the simplest and most accessible ways to use herbs. Infusions are typically made with softer plant parts, like leaves and flowers, steeped in hot water to release their properties. Chamomile tea, for instance, is commonly used for its calming effects. Decoctions, on the other hand, involve simmering tougher plant materials, like roots or barks, to extract their active compounds. Ginger decoction is widely used for digestive support and reducing inflammation.

Tinctures

Tinctures are concentrated extracts made by soaking herbs in alcohol or glycerin.

The alcohol extracts the medicinal properties of the plant and preserves the extract for long-term use. Tinctures are highly potent and effective for quick absorption, making them ideal for addressing acute issues like digestive discomfort or stress.

Salves and Balms

These are topical preparations made by infusing herbs in oil and then combining with beeswax or another thickening agent. Herbal salves are often used for skin ailments like cuts, burns, and rashes. Calendula, a popular herb in salve form, is known for its skin-soothing and anti-inflammatory properties.

Capsules and Powders

For people who prefer not to taste herbs, powdered herbs encapsulated in pills provide an easy alternative. Turmeric capsules, for example, are widely used to reduce inflammation and support joint health.

Essential Oils

Essential oils are highly concentrated plant extracts used for aromatherapy and topical applications. Lavender essential oil, known for its calming properties, is often used in aromatherapy to support relaxation and better sleep.

Each of these forms has unique applications, and selecting the appropriate form depends on the individual's needs, the herb's properties, and the desired effects.

Getting Started with Herbs

How to Source and Prepare Herbs Safely

The effectiveness of herbal medicine depends significantly on the quality of the herbs used. When sourcing herbs, it is essential to prioritize quality and purity.

These are some tips for safely sourcing and preparing herbs:

Buy from Reputable Suppliers: Many online retailers and health food stores sell herbs, but it's best to purchase from certified suppliers who specialize in herbal products. Certified organic herbs are preferred, as they are free from pesticides and synthetic chemicals.

Grow Your Own: Growing herbs is a rewarding way to ensure the quality of your plants. Herbs like basil, rosemary, and peppermint are easy to cultivate in small spaces and provide a fresh, readily available source for remedies.

Wildcrafting with Caution: Wildcrafting, or harvesting herbs from the wild, can be sustainable if done responsibly. Be mindful of local regulations, gather only in clean areas, and avoid endangered plant species.

Essential Equipment and Storage Techniques

Preparing herbs at home requires minimal equipment, but certain tools can make the process more efficient:

Mortar and Pestle or Grinder: Used for grinding herbs into powder, especially when preparing remedies like capsules or poultices.

Herb Scissors and Strainers: For chopping herbs and straining teas or infusions.

Glass Jars: Airtight glass jars are ideal for storing dried herbs and tinctures, protecting them from moisture and light, which can degrade their potency.

Storage techniques are vital for preserving herbs' effectiveness:

Store in a Cool, Dark Place: Heat, light, and humidity can reduce the potency of herbs, so it's essential to store them in a cool, dry environment.

Label and Date: Always label containers with the herb's name and date of preparation. Freshly dried herbs typically retain their potency for one to two years, while tinctures can last several years if stored properly.

Key Terms in Herbalism

Adaptogens: Herbs that help the body adapt to stress and restore balance. Common adaptogens include ashwagandha, ginseng, and holy basil.

Carminative: Herbs that reduce gas and bloating by easing digestion. Examples include peppermint and ginger.

Demulcent: Soothing herbs that coat and protect mucous membranes, often used for respiratory or digestive issues. Marshmallow root is a popular demulcent.

Diuretic: Herbs that increase urine production, aiding in flushing out toxins. Dandelion and horsetail are common diuretics.

Expectorant: Herbs that help clear mucus from the respiratory tract. Eucalyptus and thyme are known expectorants.

Understanding these terms is helpful for identifying which herbs are suited for different health concerns.

The Science of Plant-Based Healing

How Herbs Interact with the Body

Herbal medicine works through a combination of phytochemicals naturally occurring compounds in plants that have therapeutic effects on the body. Each herb contains unique active constituents that determine its medicinal actions. These can include:

Alkaloids

Compounds with potent effects, often interacting with neurotransmitters. Alkaloids in herbs like echinacea support immune function, while others, such as those in poppy, act as pain relievers.

Flavonoids

Antioxidant compounds found in many plants, flavonoids help combat oxidative stress and inflammation. Green tea, rich in flavonoids, is valued for its health-boosting properties and ability to support heart health.

Terpenes

Aromatic compounds found in essential oils, terpenes have a variety of effects, from anti-inflammatory (as in turmeric) to relaxing (as in lavender).

Saponins

Found in plants like licorice, saponins help enhance immune function and promote healthy cholesterol levels.

These active constituents interact with body systems in different ways. For example, certain herbs modulate the immune system by enhancing white blood cell activity, while others act on the nervous system to promote relaxation or reduce anxiety.

Herbs can also stimulate organ function such as liver-supporting herbs like milk thistle, which aid in detoxification and improve liver health.

Herbal Remedies vs. Pharmaceutical Options

When comparing herbal remedies to pharmaceuticals, it's crucial to understand the differences in how they interact with the body:

Single Compound vs. Whole Plant

Pharmaceuticals typically isolate a single active compound to achieve a potent effect. This focus on "single-molecule" medicine is effective for targeting specific pathways but can lead to side effects due to its potency. In contrast, herbal remedies utilize the whole plant, with all its natural constituents working in synergy.

This complex composition often results in a gentler, more balanced action, with fewer side effects.

Symptom Relief and Root Cause Addressing

Pharmaceutical drugs are often designed to address symptoms painkillers for pain, antihistamines for allergies, etc. Herbal remedies, on the other hand, aim to support the body's natural healing processes. For instance, rather than suppressing symptoms of an upset stomach, digestive herbs like ginger and peppermint help improve digestion, easing discomfort naturally.

Speed of Effectiveness

Pharmaceuticals usually offer fast-acting relief, making them suitable for acute conditions like infections or severe pain. Herbs may take longer to show effects but can be more sustainable for long-term health support. Adaptogens, for example, require consistent use over weeks to achieve optimal effects on stress resilience.

Side Effects and Safety

Pharmaceuticals can cause a range of side effects due to their targeted action on specific pathways. Herbal remedies tend to have fewer side effects, as they work with the body's natural processes rather than overriding them. For example, using willow bark (a natural source of salicin) for pain may provide gentler relief than synthetic aspirin.

Sustainability and Accessibility

The high production demands of pharmaceuticals often result in significant environmental impact. Herbal medicine, especially when herbs are grown sustainably, has a smaller ecological footprint. Additionally, herbs are often more accessible, especially in regions where healthcare access is limited.

The Essentials for Herbal Healing

Part I of this guide provides a foundational understanding of herbal medicine, emphasizing the holistic principles that distinguish it from conventional medicine. Herbal healing is a journey rooted in knowledge, connection to nature, and respect for the body's ability to heal. By learning about the types of remedies, how to source and prepare herbs, and the science behind plant-based healing, you are empowered to make informed choices that support both your wellness and the environment.

Whether you are a beginner or an experienced herbalist, this introduction to the fundamentals is your first step toward understanding how herbs can transform health naturally, sustainably, and holistically.

CHAPTER TWO

Essential Herbs for Everyday Health

In herbal medicine, a core group of herbs is often revered for their versatility and efficacy in supporting everyday health. These herbs can be powerful allies in promoting wellness, and many are readily available and easy to use. Below are some of the top herbs Barbara O'Neill recommends, each known for unique therapeutic properties and a range of applications.

Echinacea (Echinacea purpurea)

One of the most well-known immune-supportive herbs, echinacea is prized for its ability to enhance the body's natural defenses. Rich in compounds like alkamides, polysaccharides, and flavonoids, echinacea stimulates immune cell activity, making it effective for both prevention and acute care during the onset of colds and flu.

Uses: Often taken as a tincture or tea, echinacea can be used to prevent and treat colds, respiratory infections, and other illnesses.

Safety: Safe for most adults, though people with autoimmune conditions should exercise caution due to its immune-stimulating properties.

Turmeric (Curcuma longa)

Turmeric has long been celebrated in both Ayurvedic and traditional Chinese medicine for its potent anti-inflammatory and antioxidant properties. Curcumin, its main active ingredient, combats oxidative stress, reduces inflammation, and even supports joint and heart health.

Uses: Often taken in powdered form, turmeric can be added to food, prepared as a tea, or taken in capsule form to address inflammation, digestive issues, and joint pain.

Safety: Turmeric is generally safe; however, excessive use may cause stomach upset. Those with gallbladder issues should consult a healthcare professional before use.

Ginger (Zingiber officinale)

Known for its warming, stimulating effects, ginger is invaluable for digestion, circulation, and immune support. It contains bioactive compounds like gingerols and shogaols, which help soothe the digestive system, reduce nausea, and alleviate pain.

Uses: Ginger can be consumed as a tea, in capsule form, or used fresh to support digestion, alleviate nausea, and reduce inflammation.

Safety: Generally safe, though high doses may lead to heartburn or gastrointestinal discomfort. It should be used cautiously by people on blood-thinning medication.

Garlic (Allium sativum)

Garlic is a potent antimicrobial herb known for its immune-boosting and heart-health benefits. Rich in allicin, a sulfur compound, garlic can effectively combat bacteria, viruses, and fungi while also supporting cardiovascular health.

Uses: Can be taken raw, cooked, or as a supplement to boost immunity, reduce high blood pressure, and promote heart health.

Safety: Safe in moderate amounts; excessive use may cause digestive upset. Garlic can interact with blood-thinning medications, so consult a healthcare provider if you are on such medications.

These herbs, among others, can form a basic herbal toolkit for daily wellness. Barbara emphasizes using high-quality, organically grown herbs to maximize health benefits.

Herbs for Specific Ailments

In addition to general wellness, specific herbs can target particular health concerns, from immune support and digestion to stress relief and sleep. Below are some of Barbara's preferred herbs for common ailments, including suggestions for herbal combinations and formulations that enhance their effects.

Herbal Remedies for Immune Support

Immune health is foundational to overall well-being, and herbs can play a vital role in enhancing resilience against infections.

Elderberry (Sambucus nigra): Elderberries contain antioxidants and antiviral compounds that help combat respiratory infections and flu. They are often taken as a syrup or tincture to reduce the duration and severity of colds.

Astragalus (Astragalus membranaceus): This adaptogen enhances immune function and supports the body's response to stress.

Commonly used in TCM, astragalus is ideal for building long-term immune strength.

Combining echinacea with elderberry, for example, can be especially effective during cold and flu season, as echinacea bolsters immune cell activity while elderberry offers antiviral support.

Herbal Remedies for Digestion

Digestive health is central to overall wellness, as it affects nutrient absorption, energy levels, and even mental clarity. Several herbs support digestive function and address issues like indigestion, gas, and bloating.

Peppermint (Mentha piperita): Known for its soothing effect on the digestive tract, peppermint can help relieve gas, bloating, and indigestion.

Fennel (Foeniculum vulgare): With carminative properties, fennel seeds help reduce bloating, ease cramps, and alleviate gas. Fennel tea is especially beneficial after meals.

Licorice Root (Glycyrrhiza glabra): A demulcent, licorice root soothes the stomach lining and is often used to alleviate symptoms of acid reflux and gastritis.

A simple digestive blend Barbara recommends includes peppermint, fennel, and ginger, brewed as a tea to support a healthy digestive system and relieve discomfort after meals.

Herbal Remedies for Stress and Anxiety

Modern life often subjects people to chronic stress, which can impact overall health. Certain herbs known as adaptogens can help the body adapt to stress, promoting mental clarity and resilience.

Ashwagandha (Withania somnifera): Known for its ability to reduce stress and anxiety, ashwagandha is an adaptogen that helps balance cortisol levels, the hormone responsible for stress.

Lemon Balm (Melissa officinalis): This calming herb is particularly effective for reducing anxiety and promoting a relaxed state, often consumed as a tea.

Passionflower (Passiflora incarnata): This herb supports relaxation and is useful for managing anxiety and improving sleep.

Barbara suggests a blend of ashwagandha, lemon balm, and chamomile for a calming evening tea, helping reduce stress and promote restful sleep.

Herbal Remedies for Sleep

Good quality sleep is essential for health, and several herbs can support relaxation and encourage restful sleep.

Valerian Root (Valeriana officinalis): Valerian is one of the most potent herbs for promoting sleep. It helps calm the nervous system, making it useful for managing insomnia.

Lavender (Lavandula angustifolia): Known for its soothing properties, lavender is often used as an essential oil for aromatherapy to reduce stress and improve sleep quality.

Combining valerian, chamomile, and lavender in a tea can create a powerful natural sleep aid that eases the mind and body into relaxation.

Rare and Lost Remedies

Beyond these well-known herbs, there exists a range of lesser-known, "forgotten" plants with powerful healing properties. Many of these have fallen out of use over time due to shifts toward conventional medicine, but Barbara highlights their historical significance and potential to offer modern benefits.

Herbs with Historical Significance

Certain plants were revered in ancient cultures for their medicinal properties but have since become less common. Reviving these remedies can connect us to traditional practices that valued plant-based healing.

Elecampane (Inula helenium): Historically used as a lung tonic, elecampane has potent expectorant properties, making it helpful for clearing respiratory congestion and easing coughs.

Wood Betony (Stachys officinalis): Known as a cure-all in Medieval Europe, wood betony has a variety of uses, from relieving headaches and anxiety to supporting digestion.

Boneset (Eupatorium perfoliatum): Used by Indigenous North American tribes and early settlers, boneset was traditionally employed to relieve symptoms of flu, fever, and body aches.

Reviving Ancient Practices for Modern Benefits

In addition to individual herbs, ancient herbal practices emphasize the holistic principles of seasonal and natural rhythms in healing.

For example, TCM practitioners have long encouraged balancing "hot" and "cold" herbs to support the body's equilibrium. Similarly, Ayurveda focuses on the individual's constitution, or dosha, when choosing herbs.

Revisiting such approaches, Barbara advocates for using herbal remedies not only to target ailments but to align our bodies with nature's cycles. For instance, warming herbs like ginger and cinnamon are ideal in winter to promote circulation, while cooling herbs like peppermint are preferred in summer to counteract heat.

Safety and Contraindications for Common Herbs

While herbal medicine is generally safe, understanding safety guidelines is crucial. Here are some general considerations:

Allergic Reactions: Some herbs, such as chamomile or echinacea, can cause allergic reactions, particularly in individuals sensitive to plants in the daisy family.

Interactions with Medications: Certain herbs can interact with medications. For instance, St. John's Wort can reduce the effectiveness of birth control pills and antidepressants, while ginger and garlic may interact with blood thinners.

Pregnancy and Breastfeeding: Pregnant and breastfeeding women should consult a healthcare provider before using herbs, as certain plants like licorice and sage may not be safe.

Guidelines for Safe Use

Start Slowly: When introducing a new herb, start with a small dose to observe how your body reacts.

Consult a Professional: Particularly for people with chronic health conditions or those taking prescription medications, it's essential to seek guidance from a qualified herbalist or healthcare provider.

By following these guidelines, individuals can use herbs safely and enjoy their full range of benefits.

Rediscovering Plant-Based Healing for Modern Wellness

The Materia Medica is more than a list of plants it's a window into a rich tradition of plant-based healing that connects us to nature's wisdom. From common household herbs to forgotten remedies, each plant offers unique benefits that, when used responsibly, can enhance health naturally and sustainably.

Barbara O'Neill's approach to herbal medicine is about rediscovering these powerful tools, integrating them into daily life, and embracing a holistic philosophy that prioritizes long-term wellness over quick fixes. Whether you're interested in boosting your immune system, relieving stress, or supporting specific health concerns, the plants in this Materia Medica offer an accessible, effective way to support the body and soul naturally.

CHAPTER THREE

Preparing and Using Herbal Remedies

Part III introduces the hands-on world of preparing herbal remedies, emphasizing the value of making your own herbal formulations at home. Barbara O'Neill's guide to DIY herbal remedies combines the knowledge of herbalists past and present to provide natural and effective solutions. This part covers methods for making herbal teas, tinctures, balms, and tonics all practical ways to harness the healing power of plants.

Herbal Teas and Tinctures

Herbal Teas: Infusions and Decoctions

Herbal teas, or infusions and decoctions, are among the simplest yet most powerful ways to enjoy the benefits of herbs. Infusions involve steeping delicate plant parts (such as leaves, flowers, and seeds), while decoctions are suited for tougher materials like roots and bark.

Learning the right technique can maximize the therapeutic compounds you extract from each plant.

Infusion Method (For Leaves and Flowers)

Ingredients: Choose dried or fresh herbs suited to your wellness goals, such as chamomile (calming), peppermint (digestion), or nettle (rich in nutrients).

Procedure:

Place 1–2 teaspoons of dried herbs (or a handful of fresh herbs) per cup of water in a teapot.

Boil water, then pour it over the herbs.

Cover and steep for 10–15 minutes to allow the essential oils and beneficial compounds to infuse.

Usage: Strain and enjoy, either hot or cold. Many infusions can be taken daily and stored in the fridge for up to two days.

Decoction Method (For Roots and Bark)

Ingredients: For tougher plant materials like ginger root, dandelion root, or cinnamon bark, decoctions are preferable.

Procedure:

Place about 1 tablespoon of dried herbs per cup of water in a pot.

Bring to a boil, then reduce the heat and simmer for 15–30 minutes to release the active compounds.

Usage: Strain the decoction and drink. Decoctions can be added to soups or other beverages as an additional way to take your herbs.

Infusions and decoctions are an ideal starting point for newcomers to herbal medicine. They can be tailored to specific health goals, whether for relaxation, digestion, or immune support.

Tincture-Making for Concentrated Herbal Extracts

Tinctures are liquid herbal extracts made by soaking herbs in alcohol or vinegar. They are an efficient way to capture and concentrate the plant's active ingredients, making them highly potent and long-lasting remedies.

Basic Tincture Recipe

Ingredients: Fresh or dried herbs and a solvent, typically vodka (for alcohol-based tinctures) or apple cider vinegar (for a non-alcoholic option).

Procedure:

Step 1: Chop fresh herbs or grind dried herbs and place them in a glass jar, filling about 1/3 of the jar for dried herbs or 1/2 for fresh herbs.

Step 2: Pour the alcohol or vinegar over the herbs until they're completely covered and there's about an inch of liquid above the herbs.

Step 3: Seal the jar tightly and store it in a cool, dark place, shaking it daily for 4–6 weeks.

Straining and Bottling: After 4–6 weeks, strain the mixture through a fine sieve or cheesecloth, squeezing out as much liquid as possible. Pour the tincture into a dropper bottle.

Using Tinctures: Tinctures are potent, so they're taken in small doses, usually 10–30 drops in water or tea, up to three times daily. Store tinctures in dark glass bottles, and they can last for several years.

Alcohol-based tinctures are preferred for their long shelf life and ability to extract a wide range of compounds, while vinegar-based tinctures are a gentler choice for children or those who avoid alcohol.

Balms, Salves, and Ointments

Herbal balms, salves, and ointments are topical remedies that use oils infused with medicinal herbs.

They are ideal for addressing skin concerns like cuts, burns, dryness, or inflammation. Making your own allows you to control ingredients, use fresh herbs, and avoid synthetic additives found in commercial products.

Basic Ingredients for Topical Remedies

Carrier Oil: Olive, coconut, and jojoba oils are commonly used for infusions because they are stable and gentle on the skin.

Beeswax: Acts as a natural thickener, creating a firmer texture for the balm.

Essential Oils: Optional, for added therapeutic benefits and fragrance.

Herbs: Select herbs based on the intended use, such as calendula for wound healing, lavender for calming, and comfrey for promoting skin repair.

Infusing the Oil

Slow Method: Place dried herbs in a glass jar, cover with oil, and let sit in a warm, sunny spot for 2–6 weeks. This gentle process allows the oil to absorb the plant's beneficial compounds.

Quick Method: For immediate use, gently heat the herbs and oil together in a double boiler for 2–3 hours, keeping the temperature low to avoid damaging the herbs.

Making the Balm or Salve

Melt the Beeswax: In a double boiler, melt 1 ounce of beeswax per 4 ounces of infused oil. Adjust the beeswax for a softer or firmer consistency.

Mix with Infused Oil: Stir in the infused oil until fully combined. Add essential oils if desired, about 10–20 drops per ounce of salve.

Pour into Containers: Pour the mixture into small tins or glass jars and let it cool and solidify.

Application and Benefits

Balms and salves are applied directly to the skin for localized relief. Here are some common uses:

Wound Healing: Comfrey, calendula, and lavender balms can promote tissue repair, relieve pain, and prevent infection in minor wounds.

Skin Conditions: Salves containing chickweed or chamomile are helpful for eczema, psoriasis, and other inflammatory skin issues.

Muscle Pain: Arnica or cayenne-based balms stimulate circulation, relieve pain, and reduce inflammation.

The homemade approach provides a natural, effective, and chemical-free way to address a variety of skin ailments.

Natural Tonics and Elixirs

Tonics and elixirs are herbal drinks that support vitality, immune function, and overall wellness. These formulations are meant for regular use, building a foundation for long-term health rather than targeting acute issues. Barbara highlights them as an essential part of a daily wellness routine, as they provide subtle, cumulative benefits over time.

Everyday Tonics for Vitality and Immune Support

Daily tonics use mild herbs that gently support and nourish the body. They can be taken as teas, juices, or infused beverages, depending on preference.

Nettle Tonic: Rich in vitamins and minerals, nettle is a nutritional powerhouse and is particularly supportive for energy, skin health, and circulation.

Recipe: Steep 1–2 teaspoons of dried nettle leaves in hot water for 10–15 minutes. Strain and drink warm or cold.

Frequency: Daily, especially in the morning, to nourish and energize the body.

Elderberry Immune Tonic: Elderberry is known for its immune-boosting and antioxidant properties, making it ideal for cold and flu season.

Recipe: Simmer elderberries with cinnamon and cloves, then strain and mix with honey for a potent immune syrup.

Frequency: Take 1–2 teaspoons daily for immune support or increase during times of illness.

Elixirs: Combining Herbs for Unique Benefits

Elixirs are usually made by combining herbs with honey, vinegar, or alcohol. They are more complex in flavor and effect than simple teas or tonics and can be tailored to specific wellness goals.

Energy Elixir: Adaptogens like ashwagandha and Rhodiola can help boost energy, reduce stress, and improve mental clarity.

Recipe: Combine tinctures of ashwagandha and Rhodiola with a spoonful of honey and a pinch of cinnamon.

Usage: Take 1–2 droppers daily for an energizing, adaptogenic boost.

Digestion Elixir: A combination of ginger, peppermint, and fennel can support digestion, reduce bloating, and relieve indigestion.

Recipe: Infuse fresh ginger and fennel seeds in apple cider vinegar, add a few drops of peppermint essential oil, and mix with honey.

Usage: Take before meals to support digestion and prevent discomfort.

Building Routines for Wellness with Tonics and Elixirs

Integrating tonics and elixirs into your daily routine can foster long-term health benefits. Here's how to make them part of your everyday wellness plan:

Morning Routine: Start the day with a nettle or adaptogenic tonic to energize and nourish the body.

Post-Meal Digestive Aid: Incorporate a digestion elixir after lunch or dinner to support the digestive system.

Evening Relaxation: Wind down with a relaxing herbal tea or sleep-promoting elixir to support restful sleep and overall relaxation.

Each tonic or elixir is crafted to bring balance, whether by stimulating, soothing, or grounding the body. Over time, these routines contribute to a robust foundation for long-lasting wellness.

Embracing Herbal Remedies in Daily Life

Creating herbal remedies at home offers empowerment over your health and aligns with nature's gentle yet powerful healing methods. By understanding how to make teas, tinctures, balms, and tonics, you are equipped to respond to a wide range of health needs naturally and effectively.

Barbara O'Neill's approach to preparing herbal remedies combines ancient practices with practical application, making the art of herbal medicine accessible to everyone. The recipes and techniques in this section provide a hands-on way to connect with nature, support well-being, and cultivate a lifestyle that prioritizes natural healing.

CHAPTER FOUR

Herbal strategies for stress relief, sleep improvement, and mental clarity

In this section, Barbara O'Neill's Lost Bible of Herbal Remedies delves into the use of herbal remedies to address specific health concerns, emphasizing the natural support herbs offer across various systems. From immune-boosting herbs to remedies for mental wellness, this guide explains how different plants target particular functions in the body to promote balanced health. Here's a look at some of the most impactful herbal options and lifestyle strategies for immunity, respiratory health, digestive support, and mental wellness.

Immune System Boosters

A strong immune system acts as a protective barrier against infection, disease, and stressors.

Through centuries, herbalists have used specific plants known to fortify immune defenses, helping the body combat illnesses more effectively. Below are some potent immune-boosting herbs and tips for maintaining immunity.

Herbs to Strengthen and Maintain Immune Health

Elderberry (Sambucus nigra): Elderberry is a popular immune tonic, widely used during flu season to prevent and shorten illness. Rich in antioxidants, elderberries combat oxidative stress and provide vital nutrients.

Usage: Typically taken as a syrup, elderberry can be added to teas, juices, or consumed directly for daily immune support.

Echinacea (Echinacea purpurea): Echinacea stimulates immune cells and has been shown to reduce the severity and duration of colds and other infections. Its benefits come from compounds that support white blood cell activity.

Usage: Echinacea is often taken as a tincture or tea during the early stages of illness.

Astragalus (Astragalus membranaceus): In traditional Chinese medicine, astragalus is valued for its adaptogenic properties, which strengthen the body's resilience. Astragalus enhances immunity by stimulating immune cells and increasing antibody production.

Usage: Used long-term, astragalus can be added to soups, broths, or taken as a tea or tincture.

Garlic (Allium sativum): Garlic is well-known for its antibacterial, antiviral, and antifungal properties, making it an essential herb for fighting infections and supporting immune health.

Usage: Fresh garlic can be added to meals or consumed raw, while garlic supplements provide concentrated benefits.

Seasonal Immunity Tips

Increase Hydration: Staying well-hydrated helps the body flush out toxins, supports cellular health, and aids in optimal immune response.

Balanced Diet and Probiotics: Fermented foods, such as yogurt, kefir, and sauerkraut, promote a healthy gut microbiome, a crucial component of immune health.

Sleep and Stress Management: Restful sleep and regular relaxation activities, such as meditation or gentle exercise, help keep immune function strong.

Respiratory and Cardiovascular Support

Herbs that support respiratory and cardiovascular health can help prevent common ailments, like colds, while also promoting heart function and circulation. Here, we focus on plants that aid the lungs and heart, two vital systems in maintaining overall wellness.

Herbs for Respiratory Health

Mullein (Verbascum thapsus): Known for its lung-soothing effects, mullein acts as an expectorant, helping to clear the respiratory tract of mucus and congestion. It's particularly helpful during colds, flu, and asthma.

Usage: Mullein tea or tincture can be taken for relief from congestion and coughing.

Peppermint (Mentha piperita): Rich in menthol, peppermint has anti-inflammatory and antibacterial properties, making it effective for respiratory issues.

Usage: Inhaled as a steam, peppermint can help open airways, while peppermint tea soothes the throat.

Thyme (Thymus vulgaris): Thyme's antimicrobial properties make it a valuable herb for fighting respiratory infections. It acts as a bronchodilator, supporting lung health and relieving symptoms of bronchitis.

Usage: A tea or tincture of thyme helps relieve coughs, while thyme oil can be used for steam inhalation.

Herbs for Heart Wellness

Hawthorn (Crataegus spp.): Hawthorn is celebrated for its cardiovascular benefits, helping to strengthen the heart muscle, improve blood flow, and reduce blood pressure.

Usage: Hawthorn berries can be taken as a tea, tincture, or supplement, ideally under the guidance of a healthcare provider.

Garlic: Besides its immune benefits, garlic has positive effects on heart health. It helps reduce cholesterol levels, lowers blood pressure, and improves circulation.

Usage: Fresh garlic, garlic oil, or supplements are common ways to incorporate garlic into a heart-supportive routine.

Remedies for Colds, Flu, and Respiratory Ailments

Immune-Boosting Tea: Combine elderberry, echinacea, and ginger to create a warming tea that fights off infections and soothes cold symptoms.

Thyme and Honey Syrup: For sore throats and coughs, mix thyme-infused honey with warm water to coat the throat and reduce coughing.

Steam Inhalation: Using eucalyptus or peppermint oil in steam inhalation can help clear nasal and bronchial congestion.

Digestive Health and Detoxification

Good digestion and regular detoxification support overall wellness, helping the body process nutrients efficiently and eliminate toxins. Certain herbs support digestion by relieving discomfort, promoting liver health, and encouraging natural detox.

Herbal Aids for Digestion

Ginger (Zingiber officinale): Ginger stimulates digestive enzymes, eases bloating, and relieves nausea. It's highly effective for soothing an upset stomach and improving digestion.

Usage: Fresh or dried ginger can be made into tea, or added to meals.

Peppermint: Known for calming the digestive system, peppermint can relieve gas, bloating, and indigestion by relaxing the muscles of the gastrointestinal tract.

Usage: Peppermint tea is a gentle and effective remedy after meals.

Fennel (Foeniculum vulgare): Fennel seeds aid digestion by reducing bloating and gas, acting as a natural antispasmodic.

Usage: Fennel seeds can be chewed after meals or brewed into a tea.

Herbs for Liver Health

Milk Thistle (Silybum marianum): Milk thistle is renowned for its liver-protective qualities, helping the liver process toxins and repair damage.

Usage: Milk thistle can be taken as a capsule or tincture, often as part of a detox protocol.

Dandelion Root (Taraxacum officinale): A natural liver cleanser, dandelion root supports bile production and helps detoxify the liver.

Usage: Dandelion root can be prepared as a tea or tincture for daily liver support.

Detox Methods Using Herbs and Lifestyle Practices

Liver Support Tea: A mix of milk thistle, dandelion, and burdock root can be steeped into a liver-supporting tea to be enjoyed regularly.

Hydration and Fiber: Increasing water intake and eating high-fiber foods help flush toxins out of the body and keep the digestive system regular.

Sweating: Engaging in activities like exercise or sauna sessions stimulates the skin and lymphatic system, promoting natural detoxification.

Stress, Sleep, and Mental Wellness

In modern life, stress is a significant factor that impacts sleep quality and mental clarity. Herbal remedies can support the body's natural response to stress, promote relaxation, and improve sleep without the side effects of pharmaceutical interventions

Herbal Strategies for Stress Relief

Ashwagandha (Withania somnifera): Ashwagandha is an adaptogenic herb that helps the body cope with stress by balancing cortisol levels and enhancing mental clarity.

Usage: Taken as a powder, capsule, or tea, ashwagandha is typically used daily for sustained stress support.

Rhodiola (Rhodiola rosea): Known for its ability to reduce fatigue and increase resilience, Rhodiola is another adaptogen effective in managing stress and enhancing cognitive function.

Usage: Rhodiola can be consumed as a tincture or capsule, especially during periods of high stress.

Chamomile (Matricaria chamomilla): Chamomile's calming properties make it a go-to herb for reducing stress and promoting relaxation. It also helps soothe digestive discomfort caused by stress.

Usage: Chamomile tea is a gentle, soothing option to unwind at the end of the day.

Herbs for Sleep Improvement

Valerian Root (Valeriana officinalis): Valerian root is one of the most well-known herbal sleep aids, helping with both insomnia and anxiety.

Usage: Often taken as a tea or tincture before bed, valerian helps calm the nervous system.

Passionflower (Passiflora incarnata): Passionflower gently promotes sleep by reducing anxiety and encouraging relaxation.

Usage: Passionflower tea or tincture can be taken in the evening to improve sleep quality.

Herbs for Mental Clarity

Ginkgo Biloba: Ginkgo enhances blood flow to the brain, supporting memory, focus, and cognitive function.

Usage: Ginkgo is often available in capsule form and taken daily for ongoing mental support.

Gotu Kola (Centella asiatica): In Ayurvedic medicine, Gotu Kola is known for its neuroprotective benefits, aiding in mental clarity and mood stabilization.

Usage: It can be taken as a powder or tea to enhance focus.

Herbal Routines for Mental Wellness

Stress-Relief Tea Blend: Combine ashwagandha, chamomile, and peppermint to create a calming tea that supports relaxation.

Bedtime Sleep Tonic: A blend of valerian, passionflower, and a touch of honey can act as a sleep tonic, encouraging a restful night.

Herbal remedies offer a natural approach to managing a wide range of health concerns, from immunity to mental wellness.

CHAPTER FIVE

Barbara's Legacy of Herbal Wisdom

The Future of Herbal Medicine

The past decade has seen a remarkable resurgence in the use of herbal medicine, driven by a growing awareness of natural health and sustainable practices. As people seek alternatives to pharmaceuticals, herbal medicine offers a more holistic, preventative approach that aligns with the body's natural healing abilities. This movement is not only a return to ancient practices but a progressive step toward incorporating natural remedies into everyday health.

Where Herbal Medicine is Heading in the Modern Era

Modern herbalism benefits from advances in research and a more scientific understanding of plant properties. Laboratory studies have isolated and identified active compounds in herbs, validating many traditional uses.

Yet, the path forward for herbal medicine lies in balancing this scientific approach with the wisdom of traditional healing practices, which often consider the whole plant as well as the synergy of multiple plants in formulations.

Growing Public Interest and Education: With health information more accessible than ever, people are becoming empowered to learn about and experiment with herbal remedies. Courses, books, and online resources are helping herbalism reach a broader audience, bridging the gap between traditional knowledge and modern science.

Herbs in Clinical Settings: Integrative medicine, which combines conventional treatments with complementary therapies, is becoming more popular in clinical settings. Herbs like turmeric for inflammation, valerian root for sleep, and garlic for heart health are examples of remedies often recommended alongside standard treatments.

Focus on Sustainability and Ethics: With the popularity of herbal medicine rising, sustainability has become a focal point. Ethical sourcing, conservation, and cultivation are emphasized to protect the environment and ensure that wild herbs are not over-harvested.

Integrating Herbal Remedies into Your Life Responsibly

Incorporating herbal remedies into your routine requires awareness of safe practices, correct dosages, and possible interactions with medications. Here are a few guidelines:

Start Slowly: For those new to herbal remedies, beginning with one herb at a time is advisable to observe how your body reacts.

Consult with Professionals: Speaking with an herbalist or healthcare provider can help determine the appropriate herbs and dosages, especially if you're managing a chronic condition or taking medications.

Prioritize Quality and Source: Look for certified organic or wildcrafted herbs, as these tend to be higher in quality and free from pesticides.

Herbal Gardening and Sustainable Harvesting

One of the most rewarding ways to integrate herbs into your life is by cultivating your own garden. This brings you closer to the source of your remedies and allows for a fresh, sustainable supply. By growing your herbs, you can be certain of their quality, freshness, and environmental impact.

How to Grow, Harvest, and Sustainably Source Herbs

Selecting Herbs for Your Climate and Needs: Choose herbs that suit your climate, garden space, and health goals. Hardy herbs like mint, lavender, thyme, and rosemary are adaptable to various conditions, while tender herbs like basil and lemon balm thrive in warmer climates or indoor settings.

Common Herbs to Grow: Many medicinal plants are easy to grow and harvest. These include echinacea, chamomile, peppermint, sage, and calendula.

Cultivation Practices: For optimal growth, ensure your herbs are planted in well-drained soil with the right amount of sunlight and water. Raised beds or containers work well for smaller spaces, and indoor gardens are perfect for herbs sensitive to frost.

Planting Tips: Herbs like full sun, but some, such as lemon balm and mint, thrive in partial shade. Group herbs with similar water and sunlight needs together.

Soil and Watering: Herbs generally prefer soil that drains well. Overwatering can lead to root rot, so watering once the soil feels dry a few inches down is a good rule of thumb.

Sustainable Harvesting Practices: When harvesting, avoid taking more than one-third of the plant at a time to allow it to regenerate. This ensures a continual supply and minimizes the impact on the plant's health.

Wildcrafting Ethics: If foraging for wild herbs, ensure that you're gathering from healthy populations and never in endangered areas. Follow the "leave no trace" principles to preserve the natural environment.

Building Your Own Herbal Garden at Home

Starting an herbal garden can be a simple yet deeply fulfilling endeavor, whether it's on a small balcony, a backyard plot, or even indoors. This is a step-by-step guide to getting started:

Planning Your Garden Space: Choose a location with plenty of sunlight, as most herbs require at least six hours of direct sun.

If indoor gardening, consider placing pots near south-facing windows or using grow lights.

Gathering Supplies: Pots, potting soil, seeds or starter plants, and basic gardening tools are essential. Raised beds are a great option for outdoor spaces.

Growing from Seeds or Starts: Many herbs, like basil and parsley, are easy to grow from seeds, while others like rosemary and lavender are easier to start from nursery plants.

Regular Maintenance: Prune herbs regularly to encourage growth, prevent flowering (for herbs like basil and mint), and ensure the plant's potency. This step keeps your herbs in an ideal condition for use in remedies.

Harvesting and Storing: Herbs can be harvested as needed or gathered in bulk for drying. Hang herbs upside-down in a cool, dry space to preserve their potency.

Herbal gardening not only provides a fresh source of medicinal plants but also fosters a deeper connection with the plants and the earth.

Passing Down the Knowledge

One of the most profound aspects of herbal medicine is its rich legacy, passed down through generations. Sharing this knowledge, whether through teaching, written records, or community engagement, ensures that the healing power of nature endures.

Sharing Herbal Knowledge with Others

There are numerous ways to share herbal wisdom and encourage others to explore the benefits of natural remedies. Here are a few:

Teaching and Mentorship: Mentoring friends, family, or community members introduces others to the world of herbal medicine.

Workshops, online classes, and neighborhood groups create opportunities to share knowledge and inspire others.

Documenting and Writing: Recording personal experiences, recipes, and observations of herbal use creates a valuable resource. Writing articles, blogs, or even books can help to preserve and spread this knowledge.

Community Herbalism: Community gardens or herbal clinics can be a powerful way to make natural remedies accessible. By sharing plants, tinctures, and skills, a community can foster a supportive environment for natural health.

Building a Legacy of Health through Natural Remedies

Passing down a tradition of natural remedies is more than just teaching skills; it's fostering a mindset of empowerment, respect for nature, and holistic health.

Keeping this wisdom alive, you're ensuring that future generations have the tools and knowledge to manage their health naturally and sustainably.

Inspiring Future Generations: When children and young adults witness the power of herbal remedies, they gain a respect for natural health that can last a lifetime. By engaging younger generations in gardening, wildcrafting, and herbal remedy preparation, you're planting seeds of curiosity and respect for nature.

Creating a Personal Herbal Record: Developing a personal materia medica a written record of the herbs you use, their effects, and your experiences is an invaluable gift to pass down. This not only preserves your knowledge but also provides a practical guide for future generations.

Continuing Barbara's Legacy of Herbal Healing

Barbara O'Neill's approach to herbal medicine combines ancient wisdom with practical application, making the world of natural remedies accessible and effective. By embracing the future of herbal medicine, cultivating sustainable gardening practices, and passing down this legacy, we honor Barbara's contributions and ensure that her wisdom remains relevant.

Herbalism is not simply about treating symptoms; it's a way of living in harmony with the earth. Whether through growing an herbal garden, creating remedies for loved ones, or teaching others, this legacy empowers us to take control of our health and reconnect with nature's healing potential.

Appendices

The appendices of Barbara O'Neill's Lost Bible of Herbal Remedies provide two essential resources for both novice and experienced readers: a glossary of key herbal terms and an index of common ailments along with their recommended herbal remedies. The glossary helps clarify the terminology used throughout the book, making it accessible and easy to understand, while the index of ailments serves as a quick reference for finding specific remedies tailored to different health issues.

Understanding the terminology of herbal medicine is crucial for safe and effective practice. This glossary provides definitions for some of the most commonly used terms, enabling readers to gain confidence in identifying, preparing, and applying various herbal remedies.

A

Adaptogens: Herbs that help the body resist stress, balance hormones, and support overall health. Common adaptogens include ashwagandha, ginseng, and holy basil.

Analgesic: An herb or substance that alleviates pain. Examples include willow bark, ginger, and turmeric.

Antibacterial: A substance that fights bacteria and helps prevent infection. Garlic, thyme, and oregano oil are well-known antibacterial herbs.

Antioxidants: Compounds in herbs that protect cells from oxidative damage.

Herbs like green tea, rosemary, and turmeric
are rich in antioxidants.

Astringent: A substance that tightens tissues,
often used to reduce bleeding or improve
skin tone. Witch hazel, yarrow, and
raspberry leaf are popular astringents.

B

Bitter: Herbs with a bitter taste that
stimulate digestion and liver function.
Dandelion root, gentian, and artichoke are
common bitters.

Botanical: Refers to plant-based ingredients
used in herbal remedies and supplements.

Brew: A method for extracting medicinal
properties from herbs by steeping in hot
water, typically used for teas and infusions.

C

Carminative: Herbs that help alleviate gas
and bloating. Fennel, peppermint, and
chamomile are common carminatives.

Compress: A cloth soaked in an herbal solution and applied externally to relieve pain, swelling, or inflammation.

Constituents: The active components within an herb that produce therapeutic effects, such as alkaloids, tannins, and essential oils.

Cordial: A sweetened herbal preparation that serves as both a remedy and a beverage, often containing alcohol for preservation.

D

Decoction: A method of simmering tougher plant parts, such as roots or bark, to extract medicinal compounds.

Demulcent: An herb that soothes and protects irritated tissues, particularly the mucous membranes. Slippery elm, marshmallow root, and licorice are examples.

Diaphoretic: Herbs that promote sweating, often used to reduce fevers or remove toxins. Elderflower and ginger are effective diaphoretics.

E

Elderberry: A fruit-bearing plant often used for immune support, especially in cold and flu remedies.

Emetic: A substance that induces vomiting, used in cases of poisoning. Ipecac root is a well-known emetic.

Emmenagogue: An herb that promotes menstrual flow and can regulate cycles. Examples include parsley and ginger.

F

Fixed Oils: Oils extracted from seeds, nuts, or fruits, such as olive or coconut oil, often used as carriers for essential oils in topical applications.

Fomentation: A cloth soaked in a hot herbal solution and applied to relieve pain and inflammation.

H

Herbalist: A practitioner who specializes in the therapeutic use of plants to promote health and treat disease.

Holistic: An approach to health that considers the whole person, including physical, mental, and emotional factors.

I

Infusion: A method for preparing herbs by steeping them in hot water, typically used for leaves, flowers, and other delicate plant parts.

Internally: Refers to taking an herbal remedy orally, as a tea, tincture, capsule, or decoction.

M

Macronutrients: Nutrients that are required in larger amounts for human health, including proteins, fats, and carbohydrates.

Macerate: To soak herbs in a liquid (like alcohol or oil) for an extended period to extract their properties.

P

Poultice: A paste made from crushed herbs, applied directly to the skin to relieve inflammation or draw out toxins.

Phytochemistry: The study of chemicals derived from plants and their effects on human health.

S

Salve: A thick, ointment-like preparation used externally for healing purposes, typically made by blending oils and beeswax with herbs.

Sedative: An herb that promotes relaxation or sleep. Common sedative herbs include valerian, passionflower, and chamomile.

Sustainability: The practice of using resources in a way that does not deplete them, ensuring availability for future generations.

T

Tincture: A concentrated herbal extract made by steeping herbs in alcohol or another solvent, used in small doses.

Tonics: Herbs that support overall health and vitality, often taken long-term to strengthen specific body systems. Examples include nettle, reishi, and astragalus.

Topical: Refers to applying a remedy directly to the skin for localized relief, such as balms, ointments, or compresses.

Index of Common Ailments and Their Remedies

The following index is designed to be a quick-reference guide for addressing a wide range of common ailments with herbal remedies discussed in this book.

Each entry includes a list of suggested herbs, their benefits, and preparation methods, allowing readers to identify effective treatments for specific health concerns.

1. Allergies

Recommended Herbs: Stinging nettle, elderflower, and peppermint.

Benefits: Nettle acts as a natural antihistamine, while elderflower and peppermint reduce inflammation and ease nasal congestion.

Preparation: Prepare a tea with equal parts of these herbs, taken once or twice daily during allergy season.

2. Anxiety and Stress

Recommended Herbs: Ashwagandha, chamomile, and lavender.

Benefits: Ashwagandha is an adaptogen that helps the body manage stress, while chamomile and lavender provide calming effects.

Preparation: Combine these herbs into a tea blend or tincture to be taken as needed during stressful periods.

3. Cold and Flu

Recommended Herbs: Elderberry, echinacea, and ginger.

Benefits: Elderberry supports the immune system, echinacea stimulates white blood cell activity, and ginger provides warmth and reduces congestion.

Preparation: Use elderberry and echinacea in a syrup form, with ginger tea taken at the onset of symptoms.

4. Digestive Issues (Indigestion, Gas, Bloating)

Recommended Herbs: Peppermint, fennel, and ginger.

Benefits: Peppermint soothes the digestive tract, fennel reduces gas, and ginger aids in digestion.

Preparation: Brew a tea with all three herbs and consume after meals to ease digestion.

5. Fatigue

Recommended Herbs: Ginseng, ashwagandha, and green tea.

Benefits: Ginseng is energizing, ashwagandha supports adrenal health, and green tea provides a gentle stimulant effect.

Preparation: Take as a tincture or in capsule form for daily support, particularly in the morning.

6. Headaches

Recommended Herbs: Feverfew, peppermint, and willow bark.

Benefits: Feverfew is known for preventing migraines, peppermint provides cooling relief, and willow bark acts as a natural pain reliever.

Preparation: Use a tea or tincture of feverfew as a preventative, and apply diluted peppermint oil to the temples for acute relief.

7. Insomnia

Recommended Herbs: Valerian, passionflower, and hops.

Benefits: Valerian promotes sleep, passionflower calms the mind, and hops provide a mild sedative effect.

Preparation: Brew a tea or tincture blend of these herbs, taken an hour before bedtime to encourage restful sleep.

8. Joint Pain and Inflammation

Recommended Herbs: Turmeric, ginger, and boswellia.

Benefits: Turmeric and ginger reduce inflammation, while boswellia helps with joint health.

Preparation: Take as capsules or in a tea form, with turmeric added to meals or taken with black pepper to enhance absorption.

9. Menstrual Cramps

Recommended Herbs: Cramp bark, raspberry leaf, and ginger.

Benefits: Cramp bark relaxes muscle spasms, raspberry leaf tones the uterine muscles, and ginger reduces inflammation.

Preparation: Combine into a tea and consume during menstruation for relief from cramps.

10. Skin Conditions (Acne, Eczema, Rashes)

Recommended Herbs: Calendula, chamomile, and burdock root.

Benefits: Calendula and chamomile are soothing for irritated skin, and burdock root supports detoxification.

Preparation: Use in a topical salve or as a tea for internal cleansing and healing.

11. Sore Throat

Recommended Herbs: Licorice root, slippery elm, and marshmallow root.

Benefits: These demulcent herbs coat and soothe the throat, reducing irritation.

Preparation: Use as a tea, with honey added for extra soothing properties.

12. Urinary Tract Infections (UTIs)

Recommended Herbs: Uva ursi, cranberry, and dandelion.

Benefits: Uva ursi acts as a natural antiseptic, cranberry helps prevent bacterial adhesion in the urinary tract, and dandelion promotes urination.

Preparation: Drink as a tea or take in capsule form at the onset of symptoms.

Navigating Herbal Wisdom

This glossary and index are designed to empower readers with the vocabulary and remedies necessary for confidently navigating the world of herbal medicine. Understanding these terms and having quick access to remedies allows readers to treat common ailments effectively, fostering a deeper appreciation for the wisdom passed down by Barbara O'Neill and other herbal pioneers.